The Hom

How to Master Push-Ups in 30 Days

By Dale L. Roberts
©2016

The Home Workout Plan: How to Master Push-Ups in 30 Days
All rights reserved
September 29, 2016
Copyright ©2016 One Jacked Monkey, LLC
onejackedmonkey@gmail.com
All photos courtesy of Kelli Rae Roberts, June 2016
ISBN-13: 978-1539165460
ISBN-10: 1539165469

Disclaimer
This book proposes a program of exercise and nutrition recommendations. However, all readers should consult a qualified medical professional before starting this or any other health & fitness program. As with any exercise or diet program, if you experience any discomfort, pain or duress of any sort, stop immediately and consult your physician. The creators, producers, participants, advertisers and distributors of this program disclaim any liabilities or losses in connection with the exercises or advice herein. Any equipment or workout area used should be thoroughly inspected in advance as free of danger, flaw or compromise and the user assumes all responsibility when performing any movements contained in this book and waives the equipment manufacturer, makers, and distributors of the equipment of all liabilities.

Can't do a push-up?
Here's where you start!

Whether you're getting ready for a fitness assessment…
Or, you're trying to be a better version of yourself…
Learning how to do push-ups should NOT be so hard.
Yet, many sources online tend to overcomplicate the process.

How to Master Push-Ups in 30 Days gives you the exact workout plan to annihilate push-ups!

In this workout program, you'll get:

- Push-ups ideal for most any beginner
- Dozens of images to remove guesswork
- A fully customizable 30-day workout plan
- 8 simple push-ups with 6 different variations each
- Brief and straightforward instructions of each exercise
- Helpful guidelines and tips to get the most from your workouts
- And, so much more!

Discover why this home workout plan is right for you…
Get it now!

Table of Contents

Introduction

The fitness industry is ever-changing, overwhelming and an eclectic mix of contradicting theories and confusing dualities. No wonder most people looking to get into better shape become discouraged at the first sign of adversity. Trying to climb the mountain of information with little more than a few ideas is like trying to scale Mount Everest with only a pickax while wearing a light layer of clothing. Sure, you may climb to great heights, but how far can you truly go with only a few tools and a bit of determination?

"The journey of a thousand miles begins with a single step."
-Lao Tzu

Stripping down all the extra layers, I can take one exercise at a time, show its most basic form, then progress the difficulty each chapter. This way everyone can enjoy an exercise from start to finish and challenge themselves in new and interesting ways. If an exercise is too basic, then perform many repetitions of it. However, if the exercise is a challenge, continue to use it in your fitness routine until you have mastered it. If the exercise is just right, then test your ability in the next progression.

A few guidelines to remember when performing the exercise:

1. Breathe out on exertion, breathe in on the opposite movement.
2. Never sacrifice form for bragging rights. Just because you completed it poorly, does not mean you broke any world records. Believe me, it's all been done before.
3. When in doubt, try it out. You may surprise yourself on what you can accomplish.
4. If you can do it, then prove it. I'm a big proponent for high repetition exercises. Try 100 repetitions and if you are successful, please share it!

You will know when you are ready to move forward if you can easily do an exercise 15-30 times, but have difficulty completing the next progression in the series. Everyone could use these tools at some point and build a solid foundation in their fitness, so they always have something to shake up their routine. In the meantime, dig in and good luck!

Stand a few steps away from a wall, lean forward, extend your arms and place your palms flat at shoulder level onto the surface. Bend at the elbows and come as close as possible to the wall. Press through your palms and extend your arms. Be sure to keep your body straight from ankles to shoulders and rigid throughout the movement.

Remember, the closer you have your feet together, the harder the exercise is to complete. The further you separate your feet, the easier it is. Breathe in while descending, exhale while ascending.

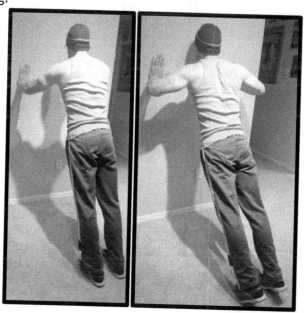

Stand a few steps away from a chair or sturdy raised surface, lean forward, extend your arms and place your palms flat at shoulder level onto the chair. Bend at the elbows and come as close as possible to the chair. Press through your palms and extend your arms. Be sure to keep your body straight from ankles to shoulders and rigid throughout the movement. Breathe in while descending, exhale while ascending.

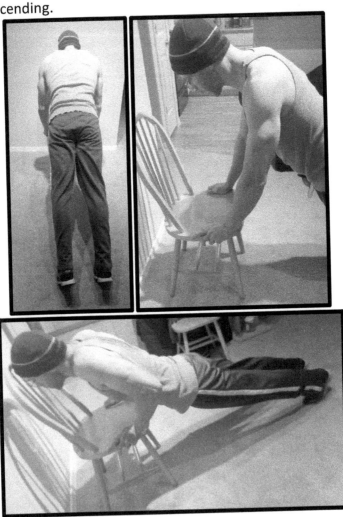

Place your knees on the ground, lean forward, extend your arms and place your palms flat on the ground. Keep your eyes focused on your fingertips. Bend at the elbows until your upper arms are parallel with the ground. Press through your palms, extend your arms and come back to the start position. Be sure to keep your body straight from knees to shoulders and rigid throughout the movement. Breathe in while descending, exhale while ascending.

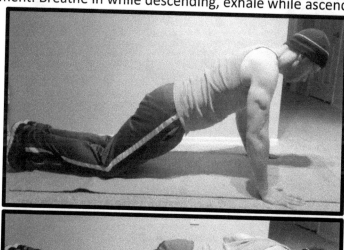

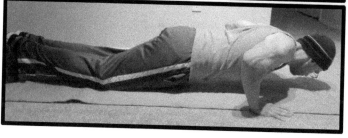

Place your toes into the ground, extend your arms below your shoulders with palms flat on the ground. Bend at the elbows until the upper arms are parallel with the floor, then press through the palms and extend your arms back to start position. Keep your vision fixed on your fingertips. Breathe in while descending, exhale while ascending.

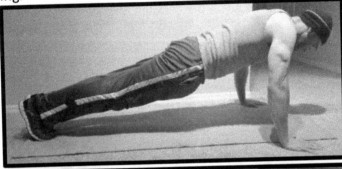

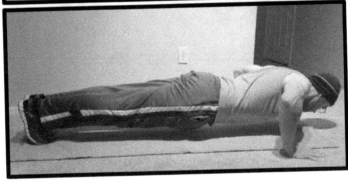

Place your feet onto a sturdy, reliable surface, such as a chair (supported against a wall) or workout bench and place your palms, with arms extended, into the ground directly below your shoulders. Keep your body straight from ankles to shoulders; ensuring your spine remains in neutral alignment throughout the movement sequence. Bend at the elbows 90°, allowing your chest descend to the floor. Press through your palms and fully extend your arms to the start position. Breathe in while descending, exhale while ascending.

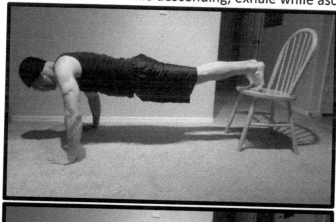

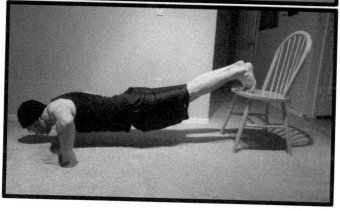

Separate your legs shoulder-width apart, place your palms into the ground about 2-3 feet in front of you and stick your butt toward the ceiling while keeping your legs and spine at a right angle from each other. In one fluid motion, dive your torso down toward your hands. As your torso reaches your hands arch upward while lifting your chin. Pause at the highest position when your pelvis is close to the floor. Reverse the movement sequence and return to the start position. Breathe in as you descend, breathe in as you ascend.

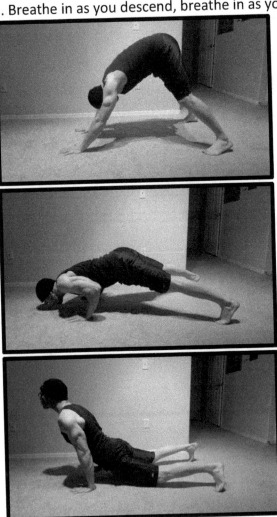

Over the next four chapters, I'm going to shift to a more difficult progression of the push-up. If you are not fully adapted to the previous exercises in this book, then do not start these exercises. I insist these next four chapters be done in sequential order since I use each chapter as a fundamental building block to performing Wall-Supported Handstand Push-ups. First, let's get you used to being head-over-heels. The blood rushing to your head can be overwhelming at first, so you need to be acclimated to this positioning before moving to the next chapters.

Perform this exercise in a clutter-free area with a thick mat until you become comfortable with it. This position leaves you a bit more vulnerable to injury if not carefully performed. Place your palms into the ground with your elbows bent at 90° and the top of your head just above (in the middle) your hands. Slowly lift one leg and place your knee on your elbow. Then, gradually lift the other leg and place it onto the other elbow. Hold this position. You should feel discomfort, but NO pain in this position. Hold this position for 5-10 seconds at first. Gradually work up to holding for one minute. When you have grown comfortable with this position, extend one leg to the ceiling and hold. Then, when you are comfortable with that position, extend both legs to the ceiling. This isometric exercise requires great balance and focused breathing. Take your time and progress ONLY when you are physically ready and able.

(see pictures next page)

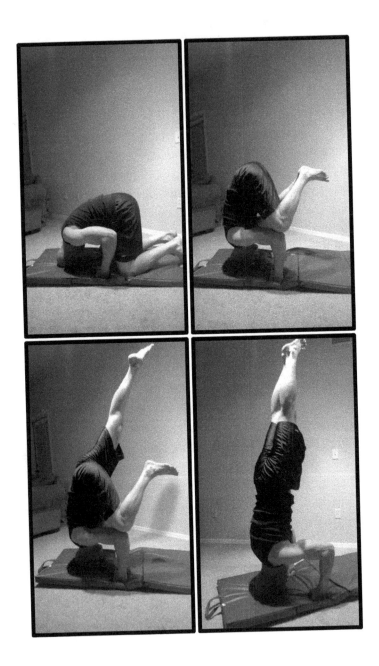

Push-up Progression 8: Wall-Supported Handstand

Once you master the Tripod, you can attempt a Wall-Supported Handstand. Get a thick mat for shock absorption, because you may come down abruptly on your first attempts. Always wear shoes for safety. When you become more practiced, shoeless is an option. Place your palms into the ground about shoulder-width apart with your fingertips about 6-12 inches from the wall. Keep your arms extended and look toward your hands. Stagger your feet, then explosively press threw the balls of your feet and aim for your heels to connect with the wall. Extend your legs and allow them to balance you with the support of the wall. Hold this position for 5-10 seconds at first. When you are finished, collapse your knees and bring your feet down toward the ground. Your first attempt may not be graceful, hence the mat and shoes for shock absorption.

If getting into the straight-arm position is too difficult, ease into this exercise by mimicking the same movement sequence as the Tripod exercise. Once your legs are balanced on the wall, slowly walk your hands to outside of your head. Return to the mat in the same sequence as listed above.

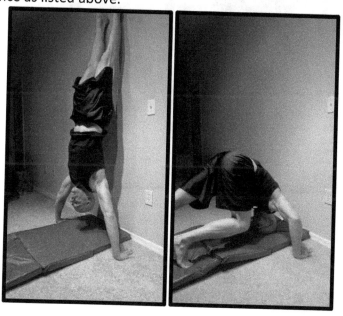

Now that you have become accustomed to the Tripod position and the Wall-Supported Handstands, you can easily perform this next movement. The purpose of mastering the previous exercises is to get you used to the blood rushing to your head. This is the closest it comes to doing Wall-Supported Handstand Push-ups. Have fun!

Separate your legs shoulder-width apart, place your palms into the ground about 2-3 feet in front of you and stick your butt toward the ceiling while keeping your legs and spine at a right angle from each other. Bend at the elbows 90° and get your head as close to touching the ground as possible. Press through your palms, extend your arms and return to the start position.

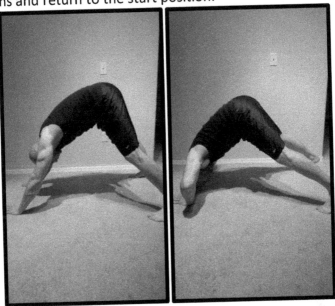

Push-up Progression 10: Wall-supported Handstand Push-up

WARNING: DO NOT ATTEMPT THIS EXERCISE UNTIL YOU HAVE MASTERED THE PREVIOUS EXERCISES IN THIS BOOK. THIS EXERCISE CAN BE DANGEROUS IF YOU'RE BODY IS NOT PROPERLY CONDITIONED OR ADAPTED TO THIS MOVEMENT.

Get a thick mat for shock absorption, because you may come down abruptly on your first attempts. Always wear shoes for safety. Place your palms into the ground about shoulder-width apart with your fingertips about 6-12 inches from the wall. Keep your arms extended, look toward your hands. Stagger your feet, then explosively press threw the balls of your feet and aim for your heels to connect with the wall. Extend your legs and allow them to balance you with the support of the wall. Bend at the elbows 90° and stop just as your head makes contact with the ground. Press through your palms and extend your arms to return to the start position. When you are finished, collapse your knees and bring your feet down toward the ground. Your first attempt may not be graceful, hence the mat and shoes for shock absorption.

As previously mentioned, if getting into the straight-arm position is too difficult, ease into this exercise by mimicking the same movement sequence as the Tripod exercise. Once your legs are balanced on the wall, slowly walk your hands to outside of your head. The difficult part is getting pushed to the top position and the first repetition is most always the hardest. Return to the mat in the same sequence as listed above.

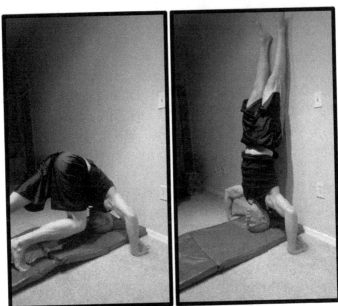

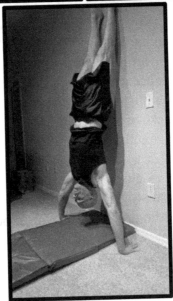

Push-up Variation 1 – Close Hand Placement

Let's add some variations to your routine and spice up the previous exercises. Ease into the earliest progression of the push-up with this new variation.

Place your hands close together on the ground. For isolating the triceps (back of the upper arm), allow your elbows to track along your ribs as you descend/ascend in a push-up. You may find some exercises harder than others to perform with a close hand placement. I find that Hindu Push-ups tend to be easier for me in a close hand position. See what is your best fit with this exercise variation. Is it Incline Push-ups with a close hand placement? Or, the Decline Push-up with close hand positioning?

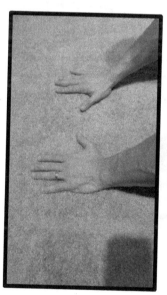
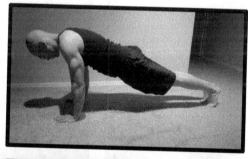
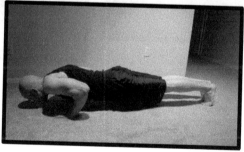

Place your hands wider than shoulder-width apart on the ground. This exercise variation can really target your chest and shoulders. You may find some exercises harder than others to perform with a wide hand placement. See what is your best fit with this exercise variation. Is it Hindu Push-ups with a wide hand placement? Or, the Decline Push-up with wide hand positioning?

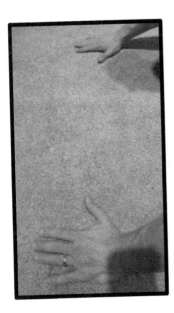
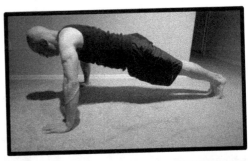
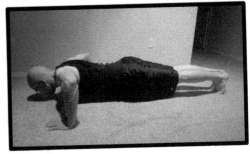

Push-up Variation 3 – Knuckled Support

Rather than using your palms for support in your push-ups, ball your hands into fists and place your knuckles into the ground. More balance is required and your forearms will light up with this variation. Ease into this exercise variation, because you may notice your knuckles get a bit raw after a few sets. Don't be surprised if you develop calloused knuckles after doing this movement consistently in your routine. Use common sense. If knuckled support isn't appropriate on some surfaces, then don't do it (i.e. slippery chairs, broken glass or pebbles). You don't have to be hardcore for this movement variation, you just need to be sensible and willing to try something different to train your body in new ways.

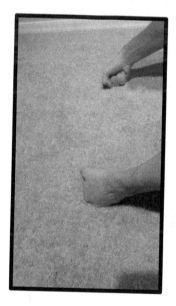
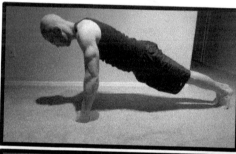
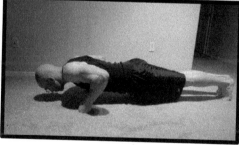

EXPERTS ONLY!

With your palms lifted/cupped, place your fingertips into the ground for support. This exercise variation is for none but the brave and is not appropriate for everyone. If you thought the Knuckled Support was tough, Fingertip Support is by far the most challenging variation. When you have mastered 5-fingers per hand on a movement, subtract a digit or two from the equation for further challenge. Good luck!

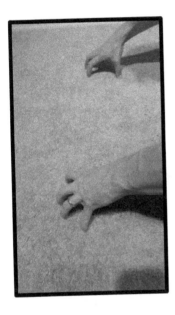
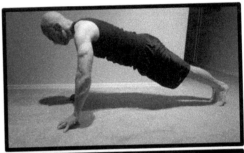
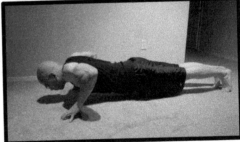

Push-up Variation 5 – Staggered Hand Placement

Place your hands shoulder-width apart on the ground with one hand slightly higher than the other. This is a great exercise for isolating one arm for training and easing into a one-arm push-up (not covered in this book). Be sure to train the staggered position equally on both sides, so switch hand positioning when you are halfway through your exercise set. Remember to use caution when trying this with the different push-up progressions as your body needs to adapt to this movement first before introducing it to more complex movements. Start with a Decline Push-up with staggered hand placement, and master that. Then, you can progress to the next variation when you are used to this new movement variation.

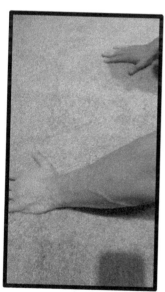
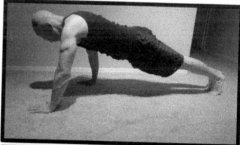
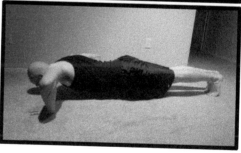

To preface this exercise explanation, it is not appropriate for all movements. I would discourage plyometrics (explosive fitness training) on Decline Push-ups with a chair for support, Hindu Push-ups and Wall-Supported Handstand Push-ups. Ease your way into this movement with Decline Push-ups with a wall. Then if you fail, the worst that could happen is you kiss the wall. And don't go all Rocky Balboa on me and start adding claps or behind the back claps; you will hurt yourself.

Choose the push-up variation best suited to your abilities. If you find a certain push-up to be challenging, then choose that variation for the entire 30 days. You'll alternate days on and off. Do as many push-ups as you can without stopping and rest for 2 minutes between 4 sets. Only do as much as your body will allow and do not sacrifice form to beat a personal record. Once you get through the entire 30 days, try to perform the maximum number of push-ups for one set to test your ability. Good luck!

Week	Sun.	Mon.	Tues.	Wed.	Thu.	Fri.	Sat.
1	W	X	W	X	W	X	W
2	X	W	X	W	X	W	X
3	W	X	W	X	W	X	W
4	X	W	X	W	X	W	X
5	X	FINAL					

W = Push-up workout; X = day off

Once you make it through the first 30 days, then try the same routine with 30 seconds of less rest time between sets. Duplicate the routine for the second 30 days, and then remove an additional 30 seconds of rest time in the following 30 days. This program will get you through at least 90 days. Once you can crank out 50-100 push-ups without rest, then you have certainly mastered push-ups.

My Thanks, Let's Connect!

Hey, thanks for purchasing my book. It means the world to me that you spent your hard-earned money and time in reading my book. I take a lot of pride in my writing, and I certainly hope you sensed that.

However, I have a huge issue I hope you could help solve. You see, I don't have a large publishing house pushing my content onto the market, in libraries or bookstores. Independent self-publishers and authors like myself rely a lot on social proof to get more valuable content published. Without some kind of third party credibility, a lot of readers would pass on the opportunity to learn the same things you have within this book.

So, could you do me the biggest of small favors? Could you leave a 100% honest review on this book at Amazon.com? Post your open and honest thoughts on the book. It'll help me improve my future releases and assist other readers in making an informed purchase.

In the event you have questions, concerns, complaints, or compliments, please feel free to contact me at any of the following:

My blog at DaleLRoberts.com

My preferred social media at
Facebook.com/AuthorDaleRoberts

Or, just hit me up at dale@dalelroberts.com.

Thanks, again, and I look forward to connecting with you!
-Dale

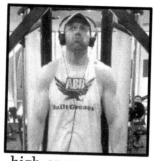

I'm Dale, a high-energy personal trainer and #1 bestselling fitness author. Today I'm in great shape, but it hasn't always been that way. I loved to read, write, and play video games, yet secretly wished to be bigger, stronger, and leaner.

Then, I discovered pro-wrestling and fell in love with the sport. The good-guy versus bad-guy stories told in the ring reminded me of superhero comics from childhood. I became motivated to push myself—to be just like those superheroes. So, I immersed myself in health and fitness information and learned to build muscle, burn fat, and develop strength. Eventually, I lived my dream of becoming a pro-wrestler and experienced some of the greatest moments in my life.

I want to share my journey—my knowledge and passion for health and fitness—and hope to inspire others into becoming the superhero they've always dreamed of being. Are you ready to become a fit and healthy superhero? Join me as I continue my journey.

Also, do you want a killer workout plan to get started NOW? Can't wait to get on the right track to becoming a fat-burning machine? Then go to http://dalelroberts.com/4minutes to join my online fitness community. And, you'll get *The 4-Minute Fat Burning Workout Plan* free!

Imagine dramatically improving employee health and fitness while increasing productivity and encouraging teamwork in the workplace.

Workouts in the Workplace

The Ultimate Practical Solutions to Improve Employee Health

with #1 Best-Selling Fitness Author Dale L. Roberts

Dale L. Roberts speaks around the world at corporate wellness meetings, business conferences, and executive retreats. Based on his series of best sellers, *The Home Workout Plan*, and on his professional experiences, Dale L. Roberts shares the incredible ways anyone can achieve their greatest breakthroughs and triumphant successes at work. And, all it takes is the proper training and cues to workout in your workplace to improve health, develop team-based skills and increase productivity.

To invite Dale L. Roberts for speaking at your next event, email dale@dalelroberts.com.

Hey, sign up for my weekly newsletter and I'll send you the best, cutting-edge health and fitness tips, unbelievably delicious guilt-free recipes, and some motivational insights to realize your greatest weight loss breakthrough yet!

Sign up here and get access TODAY!

DaleLRoberts.com/SignUp

Printed in the USA
CPSIA information can be obtained
at www.ICGtesting.com
LVHW022348030124
768109LV00042B/1492